Healthy Eating in the Natural

Marie Kingsley Murray

ii

Contents

Thanks

I would like to thank my granddaughter, Pharra. She played a key role in the production of this book with her wisdom and knowledge. Thank you Pharra!

I would also like to thank my grandson, Jordan, for his great work in the production of this book with his wisdom and knowledge. Thank you Jordan!

I would like to thank my daughter, Lydia, for all the inspirational and encouraging words she has given me. They were really uplifting. Thank you Lydia!

I would also like to thank my son, Lionel, for his participation in helping to bring publish this book. Thank you Lionel!

Finally, I would like to thank anyone else who helped me with this book whose name I have forgotten to mention. Thank You!

Preface

I was born in rural Alabama. My purpose in writing this book is to reach out to young people and illustrate to them what it was like growing up during my time compared to life today. It is such a huge difference! Some may already know about the differences from their grandparents while others may not have had that blessing. I hope that this book will enlighten you enough to where if you need a lifestyle change, you will become inspired to make one now while you are still young. As you read this book, you will learn that there are two roads but you can only follow one. One road will lead you to following the Creator and the way you were created. It is a road that will lead you to prosperity in every area of your life. The other road will lead you to destruction and as you grow older, your life will deteriorate and you will feel hopeless, weak, and useless. It is up to you to decide which road to choose. I have already learned from personal experience and I had to choose a road to take. I hope this book will enlighten your spirit and help you make wise decisions about yourself. It does not matter who you are, we can all choose which road we will follow. I hope that you will make wise decisions about your life while you are young based on my experiences and my hope is that as you read this book, something about my life will help and motivate you to start thinking about your destiny.

1

The Natural versus the Unnatural

About fifteen years ago, I started on a journey in which I was trying to connect the missing pieces that I had lost. First, I started by remembering my childhood. My thinking led me to reflect back on when I was growing up in southern Alabama on a very large farm. Many thoughts raced through my mind. I began to think about country life and city life. The more I thought about my childhood on the farm, the more I was able to compare the differences between the two lifestyles. After I had moved away from the farm during my early adult years, I lived in the city. I, however, lost something that was vital for living a healthy and joyful life. I began to realize that on the farm, everything came from the supernatural. As I continued to ponder, I realized that in order for me to live and be as healthy as possible, I needed to connect back to the natural.

On the farm, we lived based on cycles and seasons. We went to bed around eight and received a full nights rest. We woke up around four in the morning. I remember how I could always hear roosters crowing at the break of dawn and how my mother was in the kitchen every morning before the first rays of sun even hit the ground. She made a fresh organic breakfast and then she would begin on our noon dinner. My mother cooked fresh vegetables from our garden everyday. The two vegetables that I remember the most were fresh collard greens and sweet potato cobbler. I cannot remember a single day where she did not cook every meal. My mother mostly worked in the fields for an hour after she finished cooking around 10 in the morning. My father, brothers, sisters, and I were in the fields by sunrise. If it was planting season (early spring), then we planted cotton, peanuts, corn, and sugarcane. We also raised chickens, cows, and a few other animals. The cows ate green grass, which did not have any fertilizers or chemicals on it. We had not even heard of such things. Everything was of the natural. The chickens ran around all day long and the hens laid fresh eggs. We ate the eggs a lot for breakfast.

I remember my favorite seasons. The watermelon season was one of them, which was late June to early August. I remember how sweet they were and how much I really enjoyed the watermelon juice and spitting out the watermelon seeds. I really enjoyed peaches during their season which was June and July. I also enjoyed cherries, mulberries, and figs during their proper seasons. They were always grown naturally just as we were created naturally. I realized that I needed to do a complete lifestyle change.

In the city, I began to eat from grocery stores. This was during the sixties when the only food source was the grocery store. I noticed that my health was beginning to deteriorate as a result. I began to look for answers as to why I was beginning to fall apart at such a young age. I soon learned about chemical farming and the harmful toxins that were being put into vegetables, fruits, grains, nuts, and animals in order to make them grow and reproduce bigger and quicker. I learned everything about chemicals such as herbicides, pesticides, fungicides, fertilizers, and poisons. I was beginning to understand why the muscles in my upper extremities had collapsed, why doctors wanted to operate on me even though I was still in my child-bearing years, and why I had high cholesterol and blood pressure along with heart problems. It was because I had been eating unhealthy foods filled with harmful products. I had stepped out of the way God had originally created me. I was living a lifestyle that was destroying me. Everything I ate was from grocery stores which contained products that were not raised naturally. We were not created to consume so many chemicals; anytime that you step out of the image of God, you bring destruction into your life.

The animals today contain far too many hormones to make them constantly reproduce. Animals have seasons and cycles in which they naturally reproduce. Let's take a look at the chicken. It was created to go to the chicken house when darkness fell and rest. At daybreak, before the sun
rises, the rooster crows and the hens prepare to lay eggs during the day. This is the natural cycle of the chicken. I learned that the chickens and eggs that I was buying and consuming were raised unnaturally. Chickens should only lay eggs during the day; these chickens were laying eggs during the day and night. Man had discovered a way to trick chickens into believing that it was constantly day time, even at night, so that they could lay more eggs.

2

These eggs are unhealthy because they were produced in a process that did not give any regards to the natural cycles of God.

Even the water we use in our daily lives is not processed naturally. On the farm, all of the water that we used was fresh. We set up large wooden tubs in the yard to catch rain water for shampooing our hair. We also had a well where we obtained fresh water for drinking, cooking, and everything else. In the city, I got my water from the faucet. The water had to run through pipes that were full of lead and chlorine in order to get to me. I was using this water for everything!

As I continued searching, I began to compare cow's milk from the farm and cow's milk that I was purchasing in grocery stores. On the farm, we milked and feed the cows ourselves. The cows ate fresh green grass that was grown naturally and they drank water that we gave them from the well. The milk that I was buying from the grocery store was going through a process in which it was pasteurized and preservatives and calcium were added. Not to mention, the cows were eating unhealthy foods filled with toxic pesticides and other chemicals.

I decided that I needed to change the direction in which my life was going. The first thing I felt I needed to change was what I ate and drank. I had heard about organic farming but I was not really sure of what it was, therefore, I found as many materials as I could on organic foods. I learned that there are many different levels of organic foods. If the products contains at least 80% organic ingredients, than it can be labeled as organic. Products that are purely organic are labeled as 100% organic. I gradually began to change from conventional foods to organic foods. I discovered that organic was as close to the foods that I ate on the farm as I was going to get. The more I incorporated organic foods in place of conventional foods, the better I felt. I was not as tired and sluggish as I had been. I had

more energy and was more alert and happy. I had gotten up to 80% organic but my goal was 90%. I had given up all meats but fish. I soon learned that the oceans, lakes, streams, and gulfs where the fish were bred contained mercury which is a very harmful chemical that heat cannot destroy. I knew then that since the fish were not coming from a natural environment, I should not be consuming them. During this time, I also decided to give up all dairy products.

When my stomach collapsed, the doctors ran many tests on me and could not come up with a diagnosis. I went home without knowing exactly what had happened to me. I decided to give up all canned foods and eat only fresh foods from the organic sections of the grocery store. I quickly became a vegan and I felt myself gradually getting better. My stomach was no longer hurting and my upper extremities were also healing. My muscles were becoming stronger, I was sleeping better, and I was feeling better overall.

When I was growing up on the farm, I could see the sun rising in the east in the morning and the sun setting in the west in the evening everyday. I spent most of my days outside working on the farm. There was never an idle moment. We always had something to do. I loved looking at the blue sky and the moon and stars. After all of my sicknesses, I decided that I needed to change my thinking. The correct thinking would put my spirit back in its natural state. At that moment, I began to control my thinking. I began to get up early every morning, raise the blinds, and look out of the window. I felt that before or around sunrise, I was most connected to the natural. I also began to go to bed earlier so that I could receive a full night's rest. I felt great! I focused on maintaining positive thoughts that put me closer to God and everything He created.

I now had a complete change in my life. I spend my time outdoors on sunny days and I take more time to exercise. I have created a healthy and joyful lifestyle. I can truly say that stress has been eliminated from my life and I no longer have trouble sleeping at night. I wake up early every morning feeling great and ready to start my day by looking out of my window for the sunrise. My breakfast consists of a variety of fresh organic fruits, nuts, some vegetables, and bottled water. My dinner consists of a large

fresh organic green leafy lettuce salad, vegetables, and a sweet fresh organic fruit. My supper is my smallest meal. It consists of vegetables and water. I look for organic fruits and vegetables that are high in antioxidants. Before I begin my meals, I always give God thanks in prayer. I have a strong faith in God.

I have often wondered about the land and the people of the Bible. I began to study and delve deeper into the scriptures. I learned that the people of those lands lived their lives in their natural cycles and seasons. These people were vegetarians and they lived off of the land.

4

Even the Hebrews that were in bondage were vegetarians. I also learned that when they were in the wilderness on their way to Canaan, which was the Promised Land, they only complained to Moses about the lack of fruits and vegetables that had been so abundant in the land that they had left. I also learned that they were extremely wise people and they lived their lives in the natural. They followed the laws and orders of God and they looked to the Universe for guidance in when to plant and harvest by looking at the moon, stars, and sun. They lived their lives in the super natural and because of this they were very healthy and extremely wise. The Hebrews were so wise in fact that the wisdom of these people is still not completely understood to this day. If we were to follow the example of the Hebrews and return to the way we were created and God's diet for us, then we would see big changes in our lives. We have stepped out of the image of the Creator. Because we have left the image of the Creator, we have many diseases and illnesses.

In the Bible, I read about Ethiopia, Egypt, Canaan, Palestine, Jerusalem, and Babylon. I began to think about the people of these lands and what they were like and how they lived. I soon learned that these people lived their lives connected to the natural. The people of Kemet, which was ancient Egypt, were especially faithful followers of living in the supernatural. They were connected with the celestial, cosmic, and the entire Universe. Even their thoughts were of the supernatural, which were God's laws.

I continued my journey by searching for an answer as to why there is so much sickness and disease in the world. The people of ancient Egypt were very healthy. Their diet consisted of fresh fruits, vegetables, nuts, grains,
and seeds. They maintained a very healthy diet and by doing so they became very wise and skilled. They possessed more wisdom than the modern man.

The ancient people of the Bible had multiple levels of energy data. Their writing and language was of high energy data. The knowledge of the interpretation of these symbols is very powerful.

I also learned that the ancient people of the Biblical lands were capable of absorbing a broad spectrum of energy frequencies or data from the Universe. These ancient people were functioning with a

5

sixth sense which came from the Universe of multiple frequencies of deep energy levels which is needed to understand the symbols.

God's original plan for man was to live forever. He created a diet for man but man fell into the temptation of sin the Garden of Eden. Because of this, Jesus came to save man. We have been redeemed from the curse. All we have to do is have love for God and have faith in Him. I thought about the power that God gave me. It has allowed me to create a joyful life in every area of my life. It is truly wonderful because I can create my own destiny. Everything began when I changed my diet and returned it to the original diet. My mind became completely renewed. I felt the elements of intellectual power and ability. My thoughts led me to Romans 12:2 in the Bible which reads:

"And be not conformed to this world, but be transformed by the renewing of your mind."

I was also inspired by Ephesians 4:23 which reads:

"And be renewed in the spirit of your mind."

When I had returned my life back to the supernatural, I experienced the transforming of the spiritual and supernatural mind. I was ecstatic. Every morning and evening while I looking out of my window at the sunrises and sunsets, I was reminded of when I was growing up on the farm in southern Alabama. I remember how much I enjoyed looking at the sun and the moon. The full moon was so bright that it was almost like day. My parents showed me the constellations and how they were like signs. Looking out of my window always makes me feel so close to creation and the Universe.

I wanted to know more about the people of the Bible so I went to the first chapter of Daniel. This chapter discusses how Daniel and his brothers received a vegetarian diet instead of the carnivorous diet that the other men were receiving. Daniel 1:4 reads:

"Children in whom was no blemish, but well favored, and skillful in all wisdom, and cunning in knowledge, and understanding science, and such had ability in them to stand in the king's palace and whom they might teach the learning and the tongue of the children."

Babylon was famous for astrology. The Babylonians were masters of astrology. The heavenly bodies were religiously observed by Babylonian and Egyptian astrologers in the belief that the sky would tell of future events that were going to take place on Earth. Their discoveries were of great importance to everyone on Earth. The

Babylonians also followed the ways of the supernatural which led to their success.

The builders of the temples and pyramids were also followers of the supernatural ways. They constructed the temples and pyramids to line up with the Universe.

Architecture, philosophy, writings, agriculture, and many other facets of everyday life were influenced by various forms of symbolic expressions. The development of agriculture required the services of individuals who were capable of plotting the heavens and identifying the appearance or disappearance of certain stars which foretold the time and return of the annual floods. These astronomers studied the heavens over a period of generations and became well acquainted with the secret of the Universe. They discovered the movement of the stars, planets, seasons, and cycles. These people are better known as the Egyptians and Babylonians. Their wisdom was far greater than people of today because they had a sixth sense.

In the ancient times, in the land of the Bible, one of the main purposes of the education systems was to create a society where the citizens would learn and understand the relationship which existed between themselves and the Universe and everything that existed in the Universe.

Two of their main Universities were IPET and ISUT where the teachers were divided into different departments. For example, teachers of the heavens were placed into the astronomy and astrology departments while
teachers of the Earth were placed into the geography department. Teachers of the depths were in the geology department and teachers of the secret word were in the philosophy and theology departments.

These Universities were seen as mysteries by foreigners who came to the Universities in order to be enlightened by the knowledge and wisdom at these Universities. The mysterious schools and Universities were found to have very knowledgeable and wise scholars.

We must take control of our destiny by beginning with having positive thoughts. We must also learn what is good for us to eat and what is not. The Bible is our guide. Avoid foods that are not produced naturally. We also need to rid our bodies of toxins that come from foods grown using chemicals through detoxification. Try to incorporate as many foods that are labeled "organic" as possible into your diet.

Psalm 119:105 says: "Thy word is a lamp unto my feet and a light unto my path." The word is the light of my path and my salvation.

When I was younger, the muscles in my upper arms collapsed. The doctor advised me to not lift anything, even a small baby. I was on six pills a day and very uncomfortable. One of the pills I was taking was a blood thinner. This pill bothered me the most because I knew that if I cut myself and began to bleed, it would be extremely difficult to stop the bleeding. When I lived on the farm, I never had to take pills. As a matter of fact, I had never even heard of any pills except for aspirin and I don't even think I took those. I was very strong on the farm and I could lift very heavy objects. I wondered why I could no longer lift heavy objects and why I had to take so many pills when I lived in the city. I was feeling so weak and tired in the city.

I hope that you can learn from my experiences how to create a healthy and joyful life which incorporates as much as the natural as possible. The first thing that you need to begin with is the diet. Remember, you are what you eat! Food has a major effect on the body. It affects your thoughts, words, actions, emotions, everything. Eating foods containing chemicals will have negative side effects on your body. Choose whether you want to be healthy, alert, and happy or unhealthy, sluggish, and unhappy. It is your choice. I have seen both sides of the argument. When I lived on the

farm, I lived a life that was of the natural and it led me to be healthy and happy. It all started with my diet. When I moved to the city, however, I lived a life that was not of the natural and it led to destruction and unhappiness. I knew something was wrong with my lifestyle and changes needed to be made in order to follow in God's plan. This is why I am telling you to take care of your bodies now while you are young and your body will take care of you when you grow older. Eat the right foods and drink natural spring water. It will make a difference. You will become more alert and you will feel great. You will be motivated to live life to the fullest. Even your sleeping patterns will change. You may find yourself going to sleep at eight or nine o'clock at night because your body will begin to send signals telling the brain that it is tired. The brain will also send signals to the body in the morning telling it to wake up and you will find that you are more alert and refreshed. All of this happened to me so I know this from personal experience. Your thinking will line up with the natural which will line you up with the Universe. The Universe will line you up with everything that you need to know to live a healthy and joyful life.

Also, do not let negative words come from your mouth or allow people to say negative words to you. It will negatively affect your thinking and cause your mind to become unhealthy. The Bible says that whatever you think in your heart is what you become. You must have control over your environment. Be selective when it comes to picking friends. If you keep your environment in the natural, then you will know who to be around and who to avoid.

If you keep your mind in the natural, you will send wise thinking to the Universe and the Universe will send wisdom back to you. I experience this every day because of my diet. Food plays a major role in our wellbeing. It determines whether we will be healthy or unhealthy. If we begin to eliminate the use of chemicals in our foods now, then we can eliminate many of the diseases that currently plague us. Many of these chemicals will destroy us. They already destroy wildlife, the environment, the water, and the air. We, however, can change this. All we need to do is return our lives to the natural. We can create our own lifestyles by altering it to support our specific needs. Learn about yourself and what you can and cannot eat. Every one's system is not the same; what works for one person may not work for someone else. Some people are able to eat all types of foods without any reaction while others are allergic to many foods. If you are allergic to something, ask yourself if the food came from the natural or the unnatural. If it came from the unnatural, then try eating the same item from the natural and see if you still have the same reaction. You may be surprised. After you create a diet that follows the natural way everything else should fall into place. A few more things that you should avoid to stay healthy include smoking, caffeine, carbonated drinks, processed foods, leavened bread, and areas where there are many cars and trucks. Once you have completed your self-evaluation you should know what foods you can and cannot eat. If you feed your brain foods that are natural, then you are creating a brain that will be healthy. Your brain will then produce healthy thoughts. Proverbs 4:23 says:

"Keep thy heart with all diligence for out of it are the issues of life."
After you do all of this, you will have a healthy and joyful life which will be stress free. Everything that once hindered your happy and joyful life will be history. You will also know which people you can be around and you will follow your heart. I always follow my heart along with the seasons and cycles. I always conduct all of my activities during the day, like I did on the farm, which is the natural way of life. I always begin to slow down when the sun begins to set to prepare myself for a much needed rest to regain my strength and energy. God created us in his image and He requires of us to keep His laws and to live within the cycles of life. I find myself more in harmony and relaxed now that I have created a joyful life. We have the authority to create whatever life we may choose so choose a healthy and joyful life. Incorporate a healthy diet, exercise, water, sunshine, rest, and relaxation into your life. Live in the natural. Begin this lifestyle while you are still young so that you can live longer and healthier. People who have a diet that consists mostly of non organic foods, meat, and diary products need to detoxify their bodies around three or four times a month by going on an organic fast. They should eat only organic foods for the duration of their fast. Exercise regularly and don't be afraid to sweat. It is good for the body and helps to detoxify it.

If we could create a lifestyle based on the natural seasons and cycles, we would greatly help our bodies. The body would not fail us and we would live longer as a result. We need to always pray and have love because the Creator was love. We should always have faith. If we can see the benefits of serving God, the sin brought onto man in the Garden of Eden will be erased by Jesus as He came to save those that were lost and through the blood we were restored.

In our natural state of mind and thinking we do have wisdom. We can connect with God and creation. Astrologers in the ancient times used the sky to predict future events. We are connected and need the sun (vitamin D) and moon. The heavenly bodies should be religiously observed. The star Sirius is the brightest star in the sky, however, during the Biblical times, it was practically invisible except for one moment during the year at the beginning of the summer solstice. Seasons and cycles occurred because the Earth's axis tilted back and forth which changed the rays of the sun from hot to cold.

It is believed that in the beginning we abided by the natural laws but sin quickly hid the natural light of reasons. We were created in the image of God and because of that holy image we hold need to hold ourselves as the regulator of all of our thoughts and actions. We need to return to our original mindset.

Ephesians 4:22-24: "That ye put off concerning the former conversations the old man which is corrupt according to the deceitful lusts. And be renewed in the spirit of your mind. And that ye put on the new man which after God is created in righteousness and true holiness."

We were created in the natural, of God in righteousness, and in the holiness of His image.

2
Who Am I?

After learning about God's laws and orders at Creation, I knew at that point that I needed to make some big changes in my life. I knew that I needed to begin with the time I was born and where I grew up. Maybe I could find answers to all of my questions.

Around 45 years ago things began to change in my life. Everything made me miserable. Many of the foods I ate were beginning to make my stomach hurt. I felt tired and sluggish after my meals, I was having trouble sleeping at night, and I was also having nerve problems. After three decades of study, in which I had not made any progress, I decided to make some changes. I began by searching for the answer to the question, Who am I? I knew that the best way to find answers was to go to the Bible, beginning with the book of Genesis and I learned the original man was created in the image and likeness of God Almighty. It was a manner that was both pleasing to God and fit to receive the breath of life. The source of man's physical makeup was the dust of the Earth, which was created naturally with rich minerals. Man was created from natural sources (Genesis 1:27).

The natural body, which was created by God, was so intricately constructed that the use of any unnatural products becomes detrimental to life and health. It is unnatural to grow fruits and vegetables using chemicals such as pesticides, poisonous gases, etc. Garments made of natural materials such as cotton, silk, linen and wool should not be mixed with synthetic materials such as polyester and nylon. God's laws and orders enhance the health and longevity of the body. Having the right diet, along with the right lifestyle could return people to God's image. If we were to return to the diet that was originally created, which includes fruits, vegetables, nuts
12
and grains, not only would the diet nourish the body and keep it healthy, it would place us back in the position of following God's laws and orders.

God established specific laws for us. We have a specific season in which to harvest. Anytime we use other ways to grow crops that are not in season, we are stepping out of God's image which sets us up for sickness including cancer, high blood pressure, diabetes, memory loss, stroke and various diseases.

Eating the correct foods and having a healthy lifestyle will heal our bodies. We must pick and choose the correct foods to consume. Organic is the best choice. We need to keep our environment as close to natural as possible.

Jesus came to save and restore everyone. If we could return to the natural and proper ways of life, love God, and have faith in Him we will receive bountiful blessings in every area of our lives. Love, faith and obedience bring blessings. If the body is properly cared for, it is the perfect healing mechanism created by God. It can dispose of wastes without the help of laxatives and pills. The body has a defense system which will mobilize itself instantly and release antibodies which will attack and destroy any viruses as well as repair all injured tissues and organs. God originally created man to live forever; however, when he stepped out of his created image, he stepped into sickness and many types of diseases. All of these diseases are destroying the human race. In order to change that pattern, we need to change the way they think so that we can return to the original image of the Creator.

The natural rest pattern is going to bed early and rising early to begin our day with a healthy organic breakfast (see Food section). We should be ready for our day. God gave us day and night. The day is for working and the night is for resting.

There are laws for principles, building a strong character and having morals. God's laws cannot be abolished! Matthew 5:17 reads, "Think not that I am come to destroy the law, or the prophets: I am not come to destroy, but to fulfill."

Our health, life, and well-being are directly tied to the celestial bodies. Exposure to moon and sun light is essential. No one can stay imprisoned
in their home watching television and expect to become healthy. Not only does television destroy our mental well-being, it also destroys our physical well-being. If we would maintain a positive relationship with God through cleanliness of mind, body, and rest then we could become fruitful for the rest of our days. In the beginning, the Creator gave us the way of life in which we were to live. When we were

deceived by Satan in the Garden of Eden, we began to feel that we had our own mind. We did not understand that we were created in the image of God and given the "God mind." Now we find ourselves trapped in the pit which we have dug. We have to seek to understand God's divine seasons and begin to obey them. This will bring a purification of the body and mind which will allow God to return to His temple. The foods we eat determine how alert, sharp, and intelligent we can become.

Man was created from the natural. When God made man, a mist came up from the ground and wet the ground. From the mud, God created man. The water and ground had minerals so therefore man's body, which is the temple of God, was already full of minerals. God created man in His image and likeness so we are to stay connected with the Maker in every area of our lives. We were created to originally live forever and if we were to create a lifestyle according to creation then we would be healthy and have the ability to eradicate most sicknesses and diseases.

We need to reconnect back to God. First Peter 4:2 (KJV) reads:

"That he no longer should live the rest of his time in the flesh to the lusts of men but to the will of God."

The respect of God is the beginning of wisdom. It is giving credence to the way He has established His order. God has established his cycles and set times and seasons. His plans and laws are a way of life. If we keep His plans and laws then we will live forever.

There are also laws about child birth, prenatal care, and postnatal care. Judges 13:2-4 (KJV) instructs:

"And there was a certain man of Zorah, of the family of the Danaties whose name was Manoah; and his wife was barren and bore not. And the angel of the Lord appeared unto the woman; and said unto her, 'Behold, now, thou art barren and bearest not; but thou shall conceive, and bear a

son. Now therefore beward I pray thee, and drink not wine nor strong drink and eat not any unclean things."

Manoah's wife had to understand that she was going to give birth to a special child who had a special mission for God. This mission is the same for all of God's children. We are the light and salt of the Earth! The angel instructed Manoah's wife, who was a symbol of the women of God's kingdom, to beware of what she ate, drank, and thought during conception because her child was special. Women must be especially conscious of their thoughts. They need to be pure and divine. Their words carry the force of creation. Being cautious of the food we eat determines how alert and intelligent we become.

We no longer follow the way of life and God. Instead, we follow the way of Satan. If we were to maintain a positive relationship with God, we would have a complete cleaning of the mind, love and faith. The Bible says whatever a man thinks in his heart that is what he becomes. In order to return our thinking to be in line with God, we must abide by this law.

I Corinthians 6:19, 20 KJV

"What? Know ye not that your body is the temple of the Holy Ghost which is in you, which ye have of God and ye are not your own. For ye are brought with a price: therefore glorify God in your body and in the spirit, which are God's."

The body is ultimately not our own, it is a creation of God and should be held sacred for God. The body should be held in its natural state. From the moment that a baby enters the world and draws its first breath, it begins the divine cycle of worshipping the living God. As the baby nurses its mother's breast, it continues to worship God. If the mother strays from the natural cycle and begins to nourish her baby with artificial milk, she becomes guilty of leaving God's original plan for her. If a child is fed artificial products, he becomes out of touch with God. If we deviated from the perfect order of God, it places us in an unnatural state of environment. We must fear God and keep His commandments "for this is the whole duty of man" (Ecclesiastes 12:13).

The high knowledge of reality is a light on the pathway of everlasting life. Only after a cleansing within our bodies will we be ready to ingest

everything. By removing all unrighteousness, we have prepared a room for righteousness. The righteous cycles of life can never be returned to the "body" of the world until we return ourselves to the natural way of life.

Women have cycles every 28 days. A complete cycle of pregnancy is nine months; an early or late delivery can mean complications. Abortion violates the order of pregnancy. The body may experience repercussions in the form of physical and mental problems. The removal of organs is also unnatural and breaches the natural cycles of the body. It is believed that in the beginning we abided by the natural laws but sin quickly hid the natural light of reasons. We were created in the image of God and because of that Holy image we hold, we need to hold ourselves as the regulators of all of our thoughts and actions. We need to return to our original mindset.

Ephesians 4:22-24 reads: "That ye put off concerning the former conversations the old man which is corrupt according to the deceitful lusts. And be renewed in the spirit of your mind. And that ye put on the new man which after God is created in righteousness and true holiness."

If we could create a lifestyle based on the natural seasons and cycles, we would greatly help our bodies. The body would not fail us and we would live longer as a result. We need to always pray and have love because the Creator was love. Also, we should always have faith.

In our natural state of mind and thinking we do have wisdom. We can connect with God and creation. Astrologers in the ancient times used the sky to predict future events. We are connected to and need the sun (Vitamin D) and moon. The heavenly bodies should be religiously observed. Proverbs 13:20 (KJV) reads, "He that walketh with the wise men, shall be wise: but a companion of fools shall be destroyed." People are destroying themselves by acting like a "companion of fools" with the toxic poisons and chemicals that we produce such as pesticides, fungicides, herbicides, toxic gases, mercury, carbon monoxide, fluoride, fluorine, etc.

3
Picking and Choosing Your Lifestyle

There is one thing we all have in common, we were all created with a strong immune system in the super natural and we were given, by God, the authority to make our own decisions. We can also choose what we want to eat. Although God gave us our diet at Creation, he also allowed us to pick and choose the way in which we would like to live and eat. We need to find out for ourselves what foods are good for us and allow us to remain healthy. We are what we eat. Some foods that are good for others may not necessarily be good for someone else. All people, however, should eat foods that do not contain chemicals. Foods that are grown using chemicals, processed, and too many preservatives are known as "dead foods." Food has lost some of it valuable nutrients. If you feed your brain foods of little or no value, it's like feeding your brain destruction. We should know by now that destruction follows destruction. Along those same lines, righteousness follows righteousness. We can radiate love, happiness, and inspiration and from our light. We can be in Jesus and He can be in us.

It is important to love yourself. God placed into you seasons and cycles that are compatible with your thoughts, thinking, and works. I have learned to really love myself. Love brings joy into your life. Joy brings peace of mind which is excellent because it is good for sleeping and sleep is essential for a healthy immune system and the production of energy. It all stems from loving yourself. By loving yourself, you automatically begin to love others and therefore you are able to produce a healthy environment. After all, you were created in love by love. I John 4:8 (KJV) reads, "He that loveth not, knoweth not God, for God is love." You can bring sun
17
shine and joy into your life with love. When you really love yourself, you will feed your brain foods that will nourish it. If we pattern our

17

life in the order of the super natural, we can live a life of knowledge and wisdom.

America has many intelligent people who have proceeded to colleges and universities. There, they have received bachelor, master, and Ph.D. degrees. They, however, are lacking wisdom. Many people are smart but they lack wisdom. When we stray away from the super natural, we lose it.

I, personally, have experienced the big differences between regular life and the super natural. I have seen and experienced great changes in my life. The beginning of the change is when I began to feed my brain foods that were organic. My brains began to emit knowledge and wisdom. I was very cautious of the decisions I made about my life and I was extremely careful about the words I spoke. I controlled my thoughts, actions, and emotions. If you can control your mind, you can create an extremely healthy life which is full of love, faith, joy, and happiness. Try it! I have sunshine in my life everyday even when the weather does not match my heart. It is all about how you treat yourself. The Bible says whatever a man thinks in his heart is what he becomes. You are what you think and what you think can come from what you eat. If you eat junk foods, then you will have junky thoughts but if you eat wise, nutritious foods, then you will have wise thoughts. Wise thoughts lead to a life full of joy and happiness. Start enjoying life every day. Remember, we all have different needs. Be sure to find what works best for you because what works for one person may not work for someone else.

In the food section of this book, you will find some foods and an explanation of the nutrients and what health benefits to expect. This is only a short list, there are many more fruits and vegetables out there that are extremely healthy for you. If you are a meat eater, be sure to add some fruits and vegetables to your daily menu to bring out the living power of wisdom in you. We all obtain some amount of wisdom; some people have simply realized how to use it to its full capabilities.

The kind of environment we create plays an important role in our wisdom. If we create a supernatural environment in every area of our life, then the seasons and cycles and all areas of our lives will be completely in the supernatural. Proverbs 2:6-10 (KJV) says, "For the Lord, giveth wisdom; out of His mouth cometh knowledge and understanding. When wisdom entereth unto thine heart, and knowledge is pleasant unto thy soul." When we receive wisdom from the Lord, our hearts can produce wisdom which will connect us to the supernatural and it will bring us health and joy.

Remove yourself from pessimistic people. If you listen to these types of people, then you are listening to words that will destroy you, your thoughts, and worst of all, your mind. Be cautious of who you are around and who you listen to because your mind controls your health, joy, peace, and self-esteem. Avoid that type of entertainment because it could take away your healthy and joyful lifestyle. I did the same thing and I became wiser. I now have a very healthy and joyful environment. Every area of my life is filled with healthy thoughts and thinking. I have a healthy mind and speak carefully which lead to healthy actions. It all comes from what I eat. Here are samples of what I ate for each meal:

Breakfast:
- A dish of fresh fruit which may include a combination of sliced pineapple, kiwi, cantaloupe, strawberries, blackberries, blueberries, cherries, peaches, or papaya
- Fresh sweet potato pancakes with fresh mango syrup
- Fresh sliced banana sprinkled with freshly baked crushed peanuts
- A glass of fresh grape juice
- A cup of fresh hot orange tea
- A glass of spring water

Dinner:

- Fresh salad which includes chopped lettuce, tomatoes, celery, raw beets, and cucumbers. I top this with an avocado dressing.
- Lentil soup with brown rice
- Freshly cooked collard greens
- Freshly baked sweet potatoes with flax seeds
- Eggplant with yellow corn

- Unleavened golden flax meal bread
- Cooked figs, peaches, or pears sweetened with raisins
- A glass of hot orange tea
- A glass of spring water Supper:
- Fresh vegetable stew which includes rutabagas, carrots, cauliflower, string beans, celery, onions, garlic, and turnips
- Brown rice
- Fresh sweet potato bread
- Freshly sliced cantaloupe
- A glass of spring water

All of my menus vary based on the seasons. I incorporate whatever fruits or vegetables are currently in season and substitute those for ones that are out of season. As you probably noticed, my supper meal is very light and my dinner meal is a little heavier. All of my menus are made based on the natural. I never add any extra salt or seasonings and I prepare all of my meals myself. It took about a year to get to the point of cooking and eating without using extra seasonings and salt. As I eat, I think more about the health benefits than the taste and that makes it more enjoyable to eat.

I have eradicated stress and disease from my life and when you can rid yourself of all of these unnecessary problems, and then you will have created a healthy and joyful lifestyle that you can enjoy everyday. You will

become cautious of how you present yourself and you will be of great wisdom. It can really happen! I am a living example. If you start right now living your life in the supernatural, it will have a profound effect in every area of your life. That will bring more love, happiness, peace of mind, joy, health, and wealth to you. It will forever change your life because you will have a life full of joy. Start now while you're young. III John 1:2 (KJV) guides, "Beloved I wish above all things that thou mayest prosper and be in health even as thy soul prospereth." We were not created to live in sickness and poor health. We are created in the supernatural and you can start now living in the supernatural. Living in the supernatural begins with the foods you eat. You must eat foods that were produced without chemicals. If you eat the right foods, then every area of your life will follow that diet.

Some people complain that the sun is too harsh on their skin and burns them. I would like to advise these people to stop eating lifeless foods and try eating foods that are in the natural. Substitute brown rice for white rice and raw sugar for white sugar. Completely eliminate processed foods from your diet and eat foods that will enrich your pigmentation such as sweet potatoes and oranges. There are many more foods out there that can enrich your pigmentation, try a variety of fruits and vegetables and see what works for you.

Love, faith, and obedience bring wisdom and the wisdom that you will acquire will make you wise about deciding which foods to eat. Proverbs 4:17-18 (KJV) instructs, "For they eat the bread of wickedness; and drink the wine of violence, but the path of the just is as the shining light that shineth more and more into the perfect day." Eating unnatural foods is like eating the bread of wickedness and drinking unpure water is like allowing violence into our bodies which is God's temple. If the foods we eat are of the natural we can create a shining light in our life that can shine brighter every day. That light will bring us to a perfect day and lifestyle. It will ultimately lead us to a happier and joyful life. Our bodies were not created to have so many chemicals in them. We must stay connected with the magic secret of the Universe. It is essential to our well being. Begin your search now so you can begin living in the great magic of the Universe. After reading this book, I hope you will be able to step and reach out

in love and faith and begin making some changes in your life today. Try the natural, rather than the unnatural, in as many areas of your life as possible beginning with what you eat. Apply everything else that you have read in this book to your daily life and watch and feel the big and wonderful changes in your everyday life. It will happen.

4
The Maker's Foods

As we take a look at some of the foods I consumed on my journey, I can now say based on my personal experience and with certainty that if you eat the right foods from the supernatural, it will heal and restore you back to health. I'm sure you're wondering, what exactly are supernatural foods? Supernatural foods are those that are in the natural soil and environment. It means that it was grown in soil that is free of all chemicals. The foods that you can find that are closest to these foods would be the ones in the grocery stores that are labeled "organic." When I switched from conventional foods to all organic, the change really made a huge impact on my life. All of the ailments and sicknesses that I had been experiencing for many years were eradicated. I gained more energy and with all of that newly found energy, I could do other things to help me remain healthy such as exercising, running, and walking.

The foods we eat can help us or destroy us. As we look at some fruits, vegetables, nuts, beans, rice, and grains, there are some foods that should be eaten every day. They are foods that are rich in antioxidants and help build a strong immune system. Some of the foods that I personally eat everyday include green leafy foods, carrots, mangos, bell peppers, peanuts, bananas, and sweet potatoes. Peanuts along with bananas and green leafy vegetables are good for assimilation to protein and are an excellent source of the "good fat." All of these foods must be **organic** in order to see results. If we come off conventional foods and turn completely to organic, we can restore our health completely, including our thoughts. With our new thinking, we will be able to go to a new and healthier mental destination. Proverbs 6:6 says, "Go to the ant, thy sluggard; consider her ways and be wise." I have experienced a complete renewing in every area of my life,

23

including wisdom, and it all came from what I ate. Now, I really enjoy and embrace life. To young people, I would like to say start to take care of your health now! Try following these steps as closely as possible:

Work during the day and sleep at night

Exercise

Eat a healthy diet

Get plenty of sunshine

Drink lots of spring water

Get fresh air

If you can follow these few steps, you will be putting yourself in a natural state that is close to the way you were created. Please, however, be careful of the foods you eat. Study the food section of this book very carefully and find foods that will work best in keeping your body healthy, especially your mind. In addition to eating properly, make sure you get the proper amount of rest each night. It is crucial to proper brain function. Also, spend some time outdoors in the sunshine and exercising. That, along with drinking plenty of water, is also good for brain cells. If we follow these steps and create a healthy mind that can connect us back to creation, Earth, and the Universe, we will be placed into where we were in the beginning, which is where we belong.

If you simply cannot live without meat, make sure that you add plenty of fruits, vegetables, nuts, beans, and brown rice to your diet. Also, if you drink alcoholic beverages, make sure you drink in moderation. I personally do not drink alcoholic, carbonated, or caffeinated beverages but if you drink these substances, drink them lightly.

Now I will direct you in some foods that we need daily to maintain our health. Please note that there are more fresh fruits and vegetables that you can choose from but this section is a great start. I eat fresh foods from this section every day and I enjoy eating these foods because I feel as if everything else in my daily life just falls into place. It feels excellent having daily

thoughts that are centered on joy, peace, and love all day, every day. Let's start picking healthy foods that we can enjoy eating every day! We can start with a good, healthy organic breakfast that will create a healthy mind. A relaxed mind brings happiness and joy in our lives everyday.

I hope this book can make a difference in every area of your life. One of my favorite Bible verses is Jude 1:22 which says, "And of some have compassion, making a difference." My love and compassion goes out to everyone on this Earth. I hope that by sharing my experiences with health and foods, you will be able to make a positive difference in your life and that you will receive joy, health, and a peace of mind everyday.

5
Fruits and Vegetables Guide

Oranges: Oranges contain a generous amount of vitamin C, which helps ward off colds, flu, and other illnesses. It is also good for the heart. **Peaches**: Peaches contain beta carotene, pectin, potassium, dietary fiber and vitamins A and C. They can lower the risk of heart disease, high blood pressure, and even some forms of cancer. Fresh peaches are a low-calorie source of antioxidants. **Pears**: Pears contain a substantial amount of fiber, potassium, and vitamin

C. **Apples**: If eaten with the peel, apples contain moderate amounts of fiber and vitamins. **Cherries**: Cherries contain iron, potassium, vitamins C and B, and beta carotene. **Grapes**: Grapes contain iron, potassium and fiber. They have been found to be powerful as detoxifiers and also in the treatment of gout, liver and kidney disorders. Research has revealed that a natural substance, which grapes produce, can help inhibit the formation of tumors. Also, dark grape juice may be more effective than aspirin in reducing the risk of heart disease. **Figs**: Figs contain minerals and vitamins and are an excellent source of calcium. **Mango**: Mangos are very rich in vitamins C and E, niacin, potassium, iron, pectin, and beta carotene. They also cleanse the blood and contain a soluble fiber that is important in controlling blood cholesterol. **Papaya**: Papaya contains an enzyme called papain, which is excellent for digestion. Also it contains generous amounts of vitamin C, beta carotene,
26
iron, potassium and calcium. Skin, nails and hair see the largest benefits of papaya. They are also beneficial for the digestive tract. **Banana**: Banana is rich in dietary fiber, vitamins and minerals. It is especially rich in potassium and the amino acid, tryptophan. Banana helps the nerves, muscles, and lowers high blood pressure. **Kiwi**: Kiwi is extremely rich in vitamin C. It is also a good source of potassium and fiber. **Pineapple**: Pineapples are a good source of vitamin C. They contain useful amounts of vitamin B6, folate, thiamine, iron, magnesium, and soluble fiber. **Plums**: Plums are a useful source of vitamin C, riboflavin, potassium, and all of the B

vitamins. Plums also supply a useful amount of several nutrients. **Strawberries**: Strawberries are an excellent source of vitamins A and C. They also contain folate, potassium, and are high in fiber. **Avocados**: Avocados are rich in folate, vitamin A, potassium, protein, iron, magnesium, and vitamins C, E, and B6. They have more protein than any other fruit. **Green Beans or String Beans**: Green beans contain a sizeable amount of protein and fiber. They are rich in vitamin C, iron, thiamine, folate, phosphorous, and potassium. **Corn**: Corn contains an ample amount of carbohydrates. It is rich in iron, magnesium, phosphorous, potassium, folate, and vitamins A, B, and C. **Bell peppers**: Bell peppers are abundant in vitamin C, beta carotene, some B complex vitamins, calcium, phosphorus, and iron. **Collard Greens**: Collard greens are copious in vitamins (especially C), minerals, beta carotene, and phytochemicals that can protect the body from diseases. **Spinach**: Spinach contains a profuse amount of fibers, iron, vitamins C and B6, calcium, potassium, folate, thiamine and zinc. **Turnips**: Turnips contain beta carotene, vitamins and minerals which can fight off diseases. They are a good source of vitamins, calcium, potassium, and fiber. The green turnips are more nutritious than the roots. The green

tops are an excellent source for beta carotene, which is an antioxidant nutrient that the body converts to vitamin A. **Sweet potatoes**: Sweet potatoes are high in nutrition. Also, they are rich in potassium, beta carotene and fiber. They contain vitamins and minerals which can cleanse and detoxify the body and boost poor circulation. **White potatoes**: White potatoes contain complex carbohydrates, protein, and fiber. **Carrots**: Carrots contain vitamin A and beta carotene which can ward off diseases. They also help to boost bone, skin, and tissue growth. They help strengthen the immune system and assist in improving vision. **Beets**: Beets contain calcium, iron, folate, potassium, beta carotene, and vitamins A and C. Beets were used in ancient times as a medicine. **Rutabaga**: Rutabagas contain vitamins A and C and antioxidants that fight certain diseases. **Cauliflower**: Cauliflowers contain vitamin C, folate, and potassium. **Broccoli**: Broccoli contains calcium, vitamin B, vitamin C, iron, folate, zinc, and potassium. **Cabbage**: Cabbage contains vitamins C and E, beta carotene, folate, fiber, and potassium. **Squash**: Squash contains beta carotene, vitamin E, and potassium. It is also an excellent source of folate, vitamins A and C, and potassium. **Cucumber**: Cucumbers are rich in vitamins and minerals. **Asparagus**: Asparagus contains vitamin C and the antioxidant glutathione. **Celery**: Celery is rich in potassium and vitamin C. **Tomato**: Tomatoes contain beta carotene, vitamin E, magnesium, calcium and phosphorous. **Eggplant**: Eggplants contain iron, potassium, vitamin C and B and calcium. **Onion**: Onions contain quercetin, which is an antioxidant used to help ward off diseases. Onions are also good for lowering cholesterol, righting off colds, bronchial congestion, asthma and hay fever. **Garlic**: Garlic contains many vitamins and minerals and is high in antioxidants and is also one of the best ways to ward of diseases.

Lettuce: Lettuce contains vitamins and minerals, folate, iron, vitamin C, and beta carotene. **Legumes (Beans)**: Beans contain more protein than any other plant derived food. They are a good source of B-complex vitamins, iron, potassium, zinc, and other essential minerals. They are high in soluble fiber and starch. Beans are among our most nutritious plant foods. **Okra**: Okra is a good source of vitamins A and C, folate, potassium, and fiber. Okra is high in dietary fiber and is a rich source of antioxidants. **Olives**: Olives are high in monounsaturated fats which benefit blood cholesterol levels. It contains a modest, low calorie source of vitamin A, calcium, and iron. **Tomatoes**: Tomatoes are an excellent source of vitamins A and C, folate, potassium, and lycopene which is an antioxidant that protects against some cancers. Lycopene is also found in pink grapefruits and watermelon. **Leek**: Leek contains iron, potassium, folate, and vitamins C and E. **Whole wheat**: Wheat is a good source of dietary fiber, all types of B vitamins, vitamin E, iron, selenium, and zinc. **Brown rice**: Brown rice contains all B vitamins, carbohydrates, fiber, iron, and calcium. They can also ward of diseases. **Oats**: Oats contain a high amount of fiber, vitamin E, some B vitamins, iron, calcium, magnesium, phosphorus, and potassium. **Rye**: Rye contains high amounts of protein, calcium, iron, phosphorus, potassium, and fiber.

The immune system defends the body from invasions by remembering every enemy it meets. Vitamins, minerals, and protein help to keep the immune system alert. Eat plenty of fruits and vegetables, legumes, nuts, and seeds to keep the immune system at its peak.

Antioxidants: Antioxidants are found in foods such as fresh fruits, vegetables, nuts, and legumes. They help to ward off many diseases.

A vegetarian diet is an economical use of the Earth's resources. Vitamins and minerals help to keep man connected to creation. People need the sun to obtain vitamin D. Exposure to the sun enables the body to manufacture vitamin D naturally. People can achieve a balanced diet by eating ample amounts of legumes, nuts, seeds, grains, fruits, and vegeta

bles. Try to stay away from diary and use alternatives such as soy milk. Tofu, dark green leafy vegetables, seeds, nuts, and grains are rich sources of calcium, zinc, riboflavin, and other B vitamins. Vitamin D helps to build strong bones and teeth. Vitamins A, E, K, B5, B6, and C along with folate can be obtained by eating green leafy vegetables, such as collards, along with some fruits and other vegetables.

Water is essential to maintaining life. It is needed in the body to carry out virtually all of its functions. Nutrients are transported to body cells through the blood.

Try to eat onions, garlic, flax seeds, and parsley every day!

Lemons along with other citrus fruits are best known for their generous amounts of vitamin C which is an antioxidant. Vitamin C has been found to thwart many types of cancer, improve the immune system by helping to fight viruses, lower bad cholesterol and raise good cholesterol, shorten the duration of colds, and help to reduce the risk of heart attacks and stroke.

Nuts are good for the nervous system, muscles and heart. Nuts are good for the heart. They keep the blood vessels relaxed and open and nuts also help to prevent clotting. They also have unsaturated fats which have been proven to lower cholesterol. Nuts help to produce red blood cells and boost the immune system. They are an excellent source of dietary fiber, magnesium, copper, folic acid, protein, potassium, and vitamin E.

Peanuts and sunflower seeds help build the immune system, improve tissue growth and help heal wounds.

Green leafy vegetables Good for skin, teeth, bones and strengthens the immune system to fight infection and

• Tomatoes

disease. Bell peppers
Melons
Strawberries

Nuts, grains, fruits and green leafy vegetables, such as collard greens, are good for assimilating protein and fat to make red blood cells. Also, they
help to produce healthy bones, muscles, teeth. They also help to boost the immune and nervous systems.

Peanuts are a key source of the phytochemical resveratrol. Eating nuts regularly has been linked to decreasing the risk of heart disease. Resveratrol also acts as a phytoestrogen. Resveratrol may also help to protect against atherosclerosis. Peanuts contain heart healthy monounsaturated fat, vitamin E, folate, potassium, magnesium, selenium, saponins, and phytosterols. A moderate fat diet with 50% of the fat content from peanuts can lower blood cholesterol levels and can also help to fight cancer. Here are some vitamins that are rich with antioxidants:
Vitamin C
Vitamin E

• Vitamin A

Here are vitamins that build a strong immune system:
Vitamin A
Vitamin B6
Vitamin C
Vitamin D

Some fruits and vegetables are not healthy. Foods that were recreated using chemicals, such as seedless watermelons, are unhealthy. Using chemicals to kill the seeds is unnatural. Also, animals that reproduce out of the natural are unhealthy. For example, hens that are tricked into thinking that it is day even though it is night begin laying eggs not only during the day but also at night when they should be resting. The egg is unhealthy because it was produced under unnatural conditions. Hens were created in the natural to roam around during the day and to eat corn and lay one egg per day. Be careful of what you are eating because some of this food will destroy your brains and create different kinds of diseases.

If we could create a lifestyle in the natural like the ancient people in the land of the Bible, who lived their lives connected to the Creator and were very wise and healthy, then we can take our brains to a higher level. We are connected to everything on Earth and everything in the Universe.

In the ancient times, in the land of the Bible, one of the main purposes of the education system was to create a society where the citizens would learn and understand the relationship which existed between themselves and the Universe and everything that existed in the Universe and on Earth.

Eat the right foods which are those that are produced chemical free. Fresh fruits, vegetables, nuts, and grains will enhance our wellbeing. We were created with wisdom in the super natural and if we eat our natural brain foods and a variety of all different kinds of fruits, vegetables, nuts, and grains not only will we look and feel healthier but we will become wiser.

The Hebrew men in the ancient times had vegetarian diets. They were skillful in all wisdom and knowledge because of their diets. Read the book of Daniel chapter 1 verses 4 and 11-17 to find out more. When we eat the right foods we get better results. We will have a healthy immune system and brain and we will feel and look healthier. Our thoughts will develop into healthier thoughts that will work in every area of our life. We may change our environments, friends, thoughts, and speech. We will begin to question certain things. What kind of air am I breathing? How many toxins am I around? Was my home built using cancer causing materials? What kind of water am I drinking? You will notice everything around you because your brain will be healthier.

It is best to eat as few chemicals as possible. I now look for organic growers in my state and surrounding states and I visit their farms and buy farm fresh fruits and vegetables. Some growers even allow you to pick your own fruits from their fruit trees and harvest your own vegetables directly from their farms. If you can make a trip to the farm, it would be well worth it. Find some organic growers in your state or surrounding states to visit. The department that certifies organic produce should be able to help you find such growers.

In the land of the Bible, the ancient people ate fresh foods everyday which came directly from their gardens and fields. Fruits and vegetables were abundant. They had mulberries, date palms, peaches, figs, oranges, bananas, olives, mangos, and papayas. They also had pomegranates, grapes, lemons, watermelons, and various types of grains. The ancient people of the Bible were extremely wise because they fed their brains with healthy foods daily. They were full of wisdom and energy because their brains operated on a six sense. They lived their lives in the natural which was the way they were created. It is well documented that the ancient people were far more intelligent than any other people. Their intelligence was so great that the intelligence of modern man cannot come close to their intelligence. When modern people understand that "we are what we eat" and begin creating healthy food, air, water, and environments. We will see big changes in our lives. That is the good news.

Minerals are compounds that originate in the soil. The mineral content in foods varies according to the composition of the soil. People, therefore, may need dietary supplements in areas where the soil is lacking in a particular mineral. Minerals make up around three to five percent of the normal body weight.

Calcium is the most abundant mineral in the body. It weighs around 35-45 ounces in the typical adult male and 27-32 ounces in an adult female. Calcium is essential for building and maintaining strong bones and teeth which hold 99% of the body's calcium. This mineral also ensures proper nerve and muscle functions as it moves in and out of bone tissue and circulates through the body.

The human body needs numerous minerals to carry out its many vital functions. They can easily be obtained from having a well balanced diet. Man was created with natural minerals from the ground and water. In order to have a healthy and joyful life, we need to stay in a natural state in every area of life. All of the different minerals we need to maintain health should come from natural sources such as fresh fruits, vegetables, nuts, seeds, grains, beans, and spring water. As people age, they need to eat plenty of foods high in calcium and vitamin D such as green leafy vegetables and legumes.

Fiber is rich in carbohydrates. Fiber is found in fresh fruits and vegetables.

Water cushions the body cells in the form of perspiration, which helps maintain a normal body temperature. During hot and humid seasons, water is an essential body lubricant. It is vital for life. Humans, animals, and plants need water. No water equals no life. Water keeps man connected to God's creation. Calcium—Sources: green leafy vegetables such as collards, turnips, spinach, lettuce, and broccoli; seeds, nuts, and figs Calcium is essential for building and maintaining strong bones, teeth, muscles, and the nervous system. Iron—Sources: Prunes, apricots, green leafy vegetables, grains, and beans Iron is essential for healthy blood and strong muscles. Zinc—Sources: Peanuts and whole grains Zinc is essential for a healthy immune system, the brain, tissue formation, growth, wound healing, and reproduction. Sodium—Sources: Most fresh fruits, vegetables, nuts, and grains Potassium—Sources: Sweet potatoes, nuts, seeds, and whole grains Manganese—Sources: Nuts (especially peanuts), whole grains, and beans Manganese is an essential component of various enzymes that are involved in energy production. Magnesium—Sources: Green leafy vegetables, nuts, seeds, grains, and most fruits It is essential for healthy muscles, bones, and teeth for normal growth and also the nervous system. Phosphorus—Sources: Nuts, grains, seeds, most fruits and vegetables It is essential for healthy teeth, bones, and to build energy for the assimilation of nutrients such as calcium. Selenium—Sources: Fresh fruits, vegetables, green leafy vegetables, and beans Selenium is essential for protecting against free radical damage. It may also protect against cancer. Selenium is an antioxidant.

We were created with super natural minerals. If we keep our super natural bodies in the super natural state in every area of our lives we will cre

ate a lifestyle full of joy daily. We will become free of stress, depression, and anxiety. We will free ourselves of worry and we will become more relaxed, nervousness will disappear. We will begin to make wise decision in our lives daily and we will not want to put chemicals in our bodies because we will have developed healthy thoughts. We will have healthy brains and immune systems. We will not eat or drink anything that is not naturally produced. We will begin to avoid all processed foods that have been tampered with out of the natural because we will know such foods do not belong in our bodies.

We will develop a natural lifestyle where our bodies will operate on cycles such as our sleep and rest cycles.

We will be able to go to sleep at certain times without any help from other sources such as warm milk or sleeping pills. Our natural sleep cycle will not need any help. Our energy cycle will work all during our working hours. Daylight is for working and darkness is for sleep.

We will create an eating cycle of when and how much we should eat. We do not need to eat a heavy supper. Our midday meal can be our heaviest meal. You should not eat anything heavy anytime around 5:30 or 6 pm. Heavy foods take longer to digest and we need to eat foods that digest quicker and easier.

Start paying attention to the old ancient proverb, "Early to bed and early to rise makes a man healthy, wealthy, and wise" because our rest cycle will create a healthy energy cycle that will mean we have a healthy brain and immune system. A healthy brain produces wisdom and knowledge. *Proverbs 3:13 in the King James version of the Bible reads, "Happy is the man that findeth wisdom; and the man that getteth understanding."* When you feed your brain with the healthy foods that you can find, such as organic foods, you will produce a healthier you. We also need healthy unpolluted air and water. We need the sun and exercise. We are super natural people created by a God of love, in the super natural, for God is love. All of the super natural minerals such as calcium, iron, zinc, sodium, potassium, manganese, magnesium, phosphorus, and selenium make up a super natural being. We also need the amount of rest according to the way we were created to rest. Whatever amount of rest we need is

what we need to get at night which is at least seven to eight hours according to researchers.

Every so often we need to go through a detoxification process to clean toxic build up which comes from unclean air, unhealthy water, and unhealthy foods. There is one quick and simple way to detoxify our bodies and create a fresh taste and breath. Try squeezing fresh organic orange juice, grapefruit juice, and lemon juice into a glass. Then add crushed ice. If you need a little sweetener, use all natural organic cane sugar. Always drink plenty of fresh spring water.

We need to begin eating our foods in the super natural. Our brain foods are very important. We can even eradicate Alzheimer's disease because it is associated with diffuse degeneration of the brain. The good news, however, is that we can keep our brain in depth with intelligence and wisdom. All we need to do is make wise decisions about what we eat. Do not eat any and everything that looks good to you!

We need to eat foods rich in antioxidants such as: sweet potatoes, collard greens, citrus fruits, nuts, spinach, tomatoes, carrots, oranges, blueberries, blackberries, strawberries, watermelon, oranges, and mango.

Proverbs 13: 20 KJV

"He that walketh with the wise men, shall be wise: but a companion of fools shall be destroyed."

People are destroying themselves by acting like a "companion of fools" with the toxic poisons and chemicals that we produce such as pesticides, fungicides, herbicides, toxic gases, mercury carbon monoxide, fluoride, fluorine, etc.

Blueberries are good for helping to prevent eye diseases. Leafy greens, such as collard greens, are also good for preventing eye diseases.

Peanuts and sunflower seeds help build the immune system, tissue, enhance growth, and help heal wounds.

Greens, sweet potatoes, mangos, red bell peppers, and carrots are good antioxidants containing beta carotene which helps protect the immune system, bones, skin, and tissue and also improves vision.

Nuts, bananas, vegetables, and green leafy vegetables are good for assimilating protein and fat. They also help make red blood cells and improve the immune and nervous systems, muscles, and heart.

Peanuts, beans, grains, and green leafy vegetables are good for the muscles, bones, teeth, and nervous system.

Leafy greens, prunes, and beans are good for the blood and muscles.

Seeds, green leafy vegetables, and sweet potatoes contain enormous amounts of vitamin E which is good for the skin, nails, blood circulation, and maintaining healthy cells.

Citrus fruits, watermelons, strawberries, tomatoes, green vegetables, bell peppers, and sweet potatoes contain ample amounts of vitamin C. They help the skin, teeth, and bones and have an antioxidant that strengthens the immune system to help fight infections.

Peas, green leafy vegetables, sweet potatoes, figs, prunes, berries, and peanuts are good for having a healthy digestive system, the skin, blood circulation, and increased energy.

6

Sunshine

When the ancient people that lived in the lands of the Bible learned to understand the relationship which existed between themselves and the Creator, their history about themselves, how they were created, and everything on Earth and the Universe, they learned to value their great pasts and their future. They learned how to use their brains at full capacity. They operated on a sixth sense which made them full of wisdom, knowledge, and understanding because of their past history. The ancient people were so wise that modern man cannot comprehend these ancient people.

The ancient people who lived in the lands of the Bible relied on the Universe and the sun which connected them to their six senses. One component of the six sense is the great power of the sun. Sunlight is very powerful and a very important part of sunlight is its abundance of vitamin D. It plays a major role in our health. It is important for a good night's sleep in the natural and a good night's sleep is excellent and healthy for the brain. A healthy brain that can operate at full capacity will in return send good and healthy thoughts throughout the entire system. These thoughts will cause the immune system to become more alert and ready to attack any and all viruses and diseases. The brain will also send signals to give us more energy, alertness, and wisdom which will take our thinking back to the Universe where it originally came. The sun also helps lower blood pressure and blood sugar, reduce bad cholesterol, produce oxygen, and help hormones. Exposure to the sun kills bad bacteria, viruses, and other diseases. With the help of the sun, you can rid yourself of stress and control your emotions. The brain produces a chemical called melanin which runs down the main nervous system sending signals throughout the body. Every movement is controlled by this system.

38

As we learn about our history, we are also learning about ourselves. As we continue to learn to value our history, then we are learning to value our future. Genesis 2:6, 7 state: "But there went up a mist from the Earth, and watered the whole face of the ground. And the LORD God formed man from the dust of the ground, and breathed into his nostrils the breath of life: and man became living soul." When we value our future we will follow the Creator's laws and commandments. The Creator gave us seasons and cycles and he gave us our diet. Genesis 1:29 reads: "And God said 'Behold, I have given you every herb bearing seed, which is upon the face of all the Earth, and every tree, in which is the fruit of a tree yielding seed: to you it shall be for meat (food)." Also on that note, Genesis 1:14 says: "And God said, let there be lights in the firmament of the heaven to divide the day from the night; and let them be for signs, and for seasons, and for days and years." So we have already read about how we are to live in seasons and cycles in the supernatural in the spirit of the Creator. We will become more relaxed when we live our lives the way we were created. The Creator gave us our lifestyle at creation. Starting today is the beginning of a great life! Live it the Creator's way and have peace and joy daily.

978-0-595-47102-7 0-595-47102-1

IMPROVE YOUR EMOTIONS AND MEMORY THROUGH BETTER NUTRITION

Fruits and Vegetables that are Excellent for Brain Cells	<ul><li>Oranges</li><li>Berries</li><li>Leafy Greens</li><li>Carrots</li><li>Tomatoes</li><li>Sweet Potatoes</li></ul>

The Mediterranean Diet Recipe

Fresh Vegetable Stew

Ingredients:
3 Carrots, peeled and chopped
2 Stalks Celery (washed) and chopped
2 Fresh Tomatoes sliced with juice
2 Fresh Zucchini sliced
1/2 Red Bell Pepper seeded and chopped
1/2 Orange Bell Pepper seeded and chopped
1 cup washed baby Spinach - whole or chopped
1 Onion peeled and chopped
3 Garlic cloves peeled an dchopped
1/4 cup Parsley chopped
1/4 cup Basil chopped
1/2 tsp Smoked Paprika
1 tsp Oregano
Dash of Black Pepper
Pinch of Sea Salt
1-1/2 tbsp Extra Virgin Olive Oil
2 cups Water or Vegetable Stock (add more if needed)

Instructions:
In a saucepan, sauté onions and garlic in extra virgin olive oil. Add sea salt and black pepper. Cover and let stand 2 minutes, then add water or vegetable stock. Add all other ingredients and let cook on medium heat for approximately 45 minutes to an hour or until done.

The Mediterranean Diet Recipe

Healthy Collards

Ingredients:

2 bunches of Organic Collards (remove stem, wash and
  cut)

1/2 chopped Organic Onion

2 chopped Organic Garlic cloves

1-1/2 tsp Smoked Paprika

Pinch of Black Pepper

2 tbsp Organic Extra Virgin Olive Oil

1 cup Water

Sea Salt to taste

Instructions:

Place onion, garlic, paprika, pepper, salt and olive oil in a
boiler, and sauté. Add 1 cup of water, bring to a boil.
Then add collards. Collards should never be covered with
water while cooking. Water should always be as little as
possible to cook until done. When collards are finished
add more olive oil if desired.

The Mediterranean Diet Recipe

The Quick and Easy Way to Detox

Ingredients:

1 Papaya

2 cups Dark Grapes

Instructions:

Peel papaya, cut in half. With dark grapes slice and remove seeds. Add papaya and grapes to juicer. Add room temperature bottled water. Blend and juice. Should be drank before a light breakfast.

The Mediterranean Diet Recipe

Mediterranean Spring Salad

Ingredients for Salad:

3 cups chopped green leafy Lettuce

1 Tomato sliced

2 Radishes sliced

1 quart Red Onion sliced

1 Green Onion sliced

1/4 cup Black Olives sliced

1 tsp baked Sunflower Seeds

1/4 cup Honey Baked Pecans chopped

Ingredients for Dressing:

1/2 tsp Vegan Worcestershire Sauce

1 tbsp Lemon Juice

6 tbsp Extra Virgin Olive Oil

Instructions:

Add salad ingredients and toss with dressing. Add sea salt and pepper to taste.

The Mediterranean Diet Recipe

Honeyed Carrots

Ingredients:

6 to 8 Carrots peeled and sliced

1-1/2 fresh Lemon Juice

1/2 cup Honey

Lemon Zest (optional)

Instructions:

Peel carrots and slice. Boil carrots in water until approximately 7 to 8 minutes (almost done). Drain water. Add juice from lemons and honey. Continue to simmer until tender.